From
Pea to Pumpkin

A Pregnancy Journal

GERALYN BRODER MURRAY

sourcebooks

Everything I do is for Chris, Reese, and Finn.
With all my love.

Published by Sourcebooks, Inc.
P.O. Box 4410, Naperville, Illinois 60567-4410
(630) 961-3900
Fax: (630) 961-2168
www.sourcebooks.com

Printed and bound in China.
OGP 10 9 8 7 6 5 4 3 2 1

This journal chronicles the progress of
_____'s little pumpkin.

ACKNOWLEDGMENTS

This little journal wouldn't have happened without:

- C, R & F
- Uncle B & Aunt C
- My mom
- My sister
- The Murray/ Carranchos
- Darcey Sell
- Dan Lazar
- The good folks at Sourcebooks
- My Dad's voice in my head: "Go with your strength."
- Chocolate
- A great deal of produce, pens, good paper, and watercolor
- Dear friends
- Dear friends with children who are friends of my children
- My animals
- Love
- Luck
- Family
- Failure
- Humility
- Gratitude
- Work ethic
- Loving where I live
- Learning how to draw (kind of) at age 40

WHY *FROM PEA TO PUMPKIN* WAS BORN

This is what I remember from ten years ago, when I was pregnant with my daughter: I craved fruit and was ill every day from week six to week ten. With my son, seven years ago, I remember that I was never ill, but instead simply bone tired, my patience short and my stomach enormous.

I know that with each of them, I was scared and elated, both.

I wish I remembered more.

That is why I created this little book. For you: so that you will have something to help you record all the little moments—and big moments—over these next nine (ten?) months. So you will have the chance to write down what you want for your child before you meet him or her, before their wonderful inclinations shape your expectations and modify your dreams with reality. This book exists so that one day, when you have a few precious spare moments, you can look back at your hopes and plans for your child before they were tethered to an actual person, when it was all only possibility.

The size of your baby each week in these pages is only approximate: one mother's papaya is another mama's peach. I'm no doctor or scientist; the produce is simply to give you a fun idea of how your sweet one is coming along.

This journal is for you and for your little pea (soon to be your little pumpkin). May every week bring you and your baby closer to health and happiness, closer to discovering all the love and simple pleasures you'll have a lifetime to share.

We're having a baby!

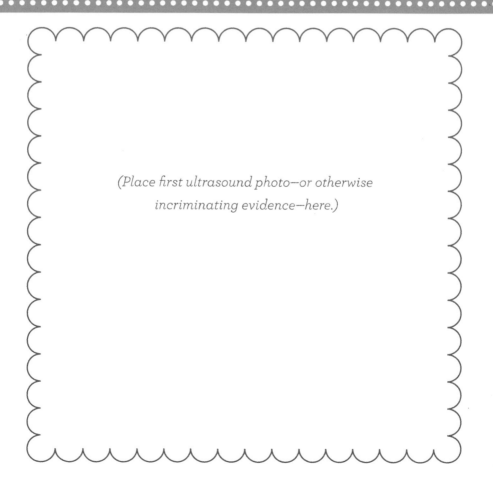

(Place first ultrasound photo—or otherwise incriminating evidence—here.)

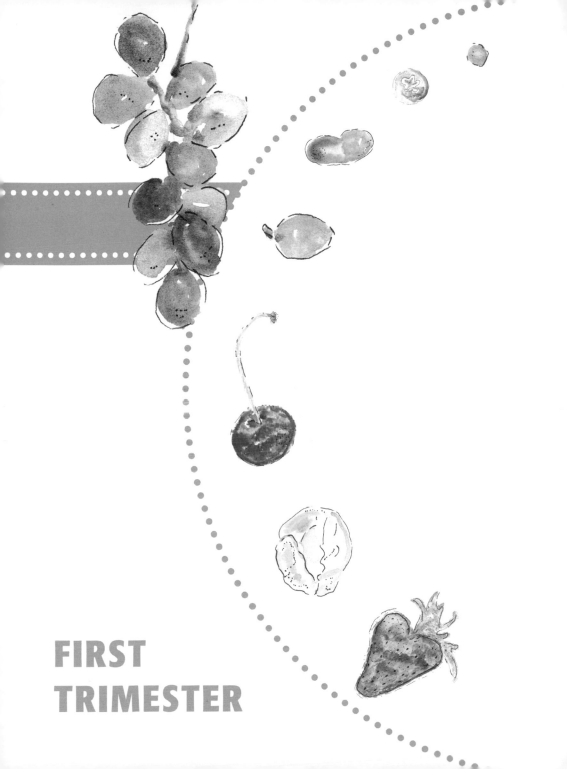

FIRST TRIMESTER

Week 6

Pea
.25 inches

WEEK 6

Right now, being pregnant seems (check what applies):

- ○ Too good to be true
- ○ Totally like winning the lottery
- ○ The scariest thing that has ever happened to me
- ○ Completely unreal
- ○ Other: _____

The thought of _____
makes me _____.
What sounds really good is _____.
My partner couldn't be more _____ _____
_____ right now.
I want _____
_____ more than I ever have.
Baby, as we begin this thing, I need you to know that _____

_____
_____
_____
_____
_____
_____
_____
_____
_____
_____.

Week 7

Blueberry

.51 inches

WEEK 7

At this point, sleep is (check what applies):

- ○ Constantly beckoning
- ○ Non-existent
- ○ Fitful. And quite uncomfortable.
- ○ Full of really bizarre dreams, involving food or attractive movie stars
- ○ Other: _____

I wish I had more _____ right now. Oh, and
_____
_____ too.
The one thing that keeps running through my head is _____
_____
_____.

I cannot wait to tell _____
_____ about this baby. And I wish I could tell _____
_____.

Baby, this week, I want you to know how much I believe in ___
_____
_____
_____
_____
_____
_____.

Week 8

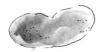

Kidney bean
.63 inches

WEEK 8

My boobs are (check what applies):

- ○ A teenage boy's dream
- ○ A bit in the way
- ○ Totally painful and huge
- ○ Lovely. Really lovely.
- ○ Other: _____

What I can't wait for is _____. And ____ ____
_____.

There is a person growing inside me. This is a(n) _____
_____ proposition.

The thing I already miss most about my pre-pregnancy body is
_____
_____.

Baby, one day, when you're old enough to read this, even thought it might seem silly, I want you to know I was scared of

_____
_____
_____
_____
_____
_____
_____
_____
_____.

Week 9

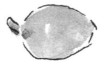

Grape

.9 inches

WEEK 9

My moods of late resemble (check what applies):
- ○ A roller coaster
- ○ A wet blanket
- ○ Those of a person I'd rather not know
- ○ Truthfully, I'm kind of a peach
- ○ Other: _____

Nausea is so _____. The one thing I'm really fortunate for with that whole thing is _____

_____

_____

When I'm away from home, I want to _____. And, when I get home, the first thing I do is _____ and, of course _____

_____

My belly right now looks _____

_____

_____

Baby, this week, one thing that's happening in the world right now that I think you should know about is _____

_____

_____

And this is how I feel about it: _____

_____

Week 10

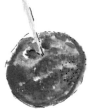

Cherry
1.2 inches

WEEK 10

Maternity clothes remind me (check what applies):
- ○ That I can make anything look good
- ○ That there will be some temporary non-hotness
- ○ That I might never feel sexy again
- ○ That elastic waistbands are a pretty great idea
- ○ Other: _____

I feel _____ _____ _____.

The thing that helps most is __ _____.

And maybe _____ _____
_____ _____.

I never thought being pregnant would be this ____ _____
___ _____ _____ _____.

I'm becoming a mother in 30 weeks. This brings to mind
visions of __ _____
_____ _____
___ _____ _____.

Baby, we plan on being the kind of parents who _____
_____
_____
_____
_____
_____
_____
_____.

Week 11

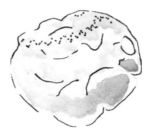

Brussels sprout
1.6 inches

WEEK 11

Lately, what's making me uncomfortable is (check what applies):

- ○ Digestion-related
- ○ Nausea-related
- ○ Clothing-related
- ○ Related to the fact that my body seems to belong to someone else
- ○ Other: _____

I cry _____. And I get emotional about _____. Or just _____ _____.

Weight gain seems _____.

The sweetest compliment I've gotten lately _____ _____ _____.

One way I've probably already messed this baby up is by _____ _____.

Baby, if you are a boy, I hope you will always _____ _____ _____ _____ _____.

Week 12

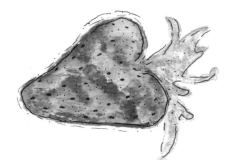

Strawberry

.49 ounces

WEEK 12

My attempt to eat well is going (check what applies):

○ Pretty well. I haven't had a French fry in weeks.

○ Hit or miss

○ I'm devouring everything in sight, and I'm OK with that

○ Mostly good with a chance of M&M's

○ Other: _____

My tiredness on a scale of 1–10 is a _____. But at night, it's more like a _____ .

I keep dreaming the baby is a _____.

Or maybe a _____

_____

So far, my favorite thing about this pregnancy is _____

_____ .

Baby, if you are a girl, I hope you always _____

_____

_____

_____

_____

_____

_____

_____

_____ .

A Pumpkin in Progress

*Use these pages to write down a story
or place a keepsake from your pregnancy so far.*

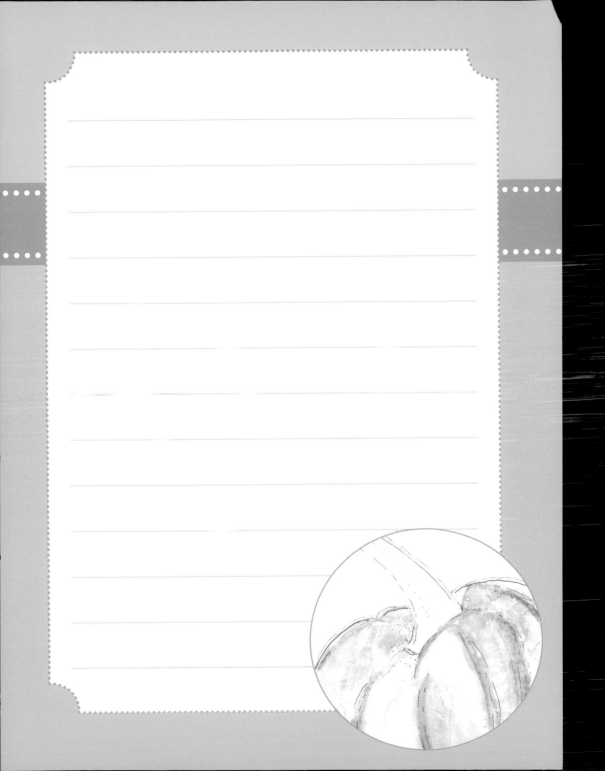

There's really a baby in there.

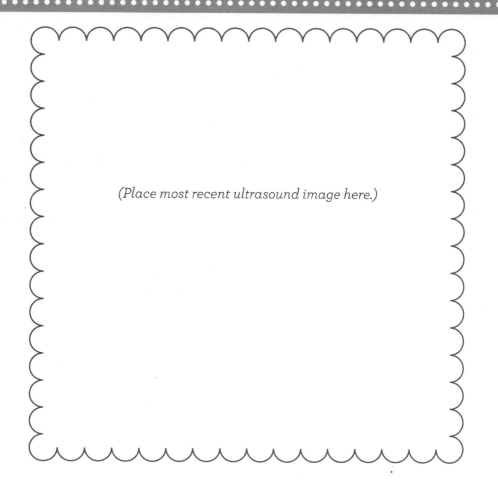

(Place most recent ultrasound image here.)

SECOND
TRIMESTER

Week 13

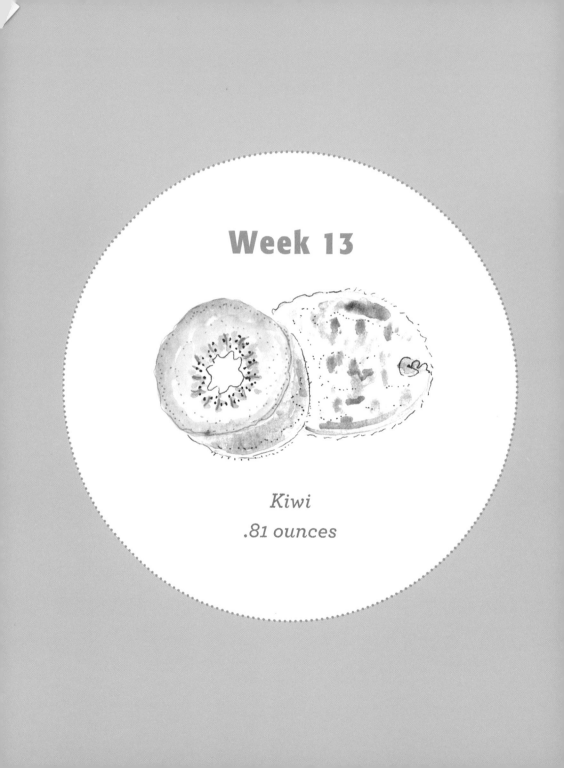

Kiwi

.81 ounces

WEEK 13

I really miss (check what applies):

- ○ Sushi
- ○ Caffeine
- ○ Beer
- ○ Other: _____

The most challenging pregnancy symptom for me is _____
_____. The one thing I'm glad
hasn't happened is _____
_____.

I'm spending most of my extra cash these days on _____
_____.

The one thing my partner and I want to do differently as
parents is _____.
Here's how we think we might work that out: _____
_____
_____
_____.

Baby, this week I want you to know about what kind of kid I was.
The truth is, I was really _____
and also kind of _____
_____
_____
_____.

Week 14

Lime

1.5 ounces

WEEK 14

I am showing (check what applies):
- ○ A little
- ○ A lot
- ○ Just enough so that people are looking at me oddly
- ○ Not at all. Flat as a board.
- ○ Other: _____

My feeling about finding out the sex of the baby is
_____.

My partner feels _____
_____. I think we'll _____
_____.

The best thing about being in the second trimester is _____
_____. And
_____, too.

As for morning sickness, it's _____
_____.

When I imagine this baby, I'm seeing _____ eyes and
_____ hair. And a disposition like his/her _____
_____.

Baby, you should know this about your grandparents: _____
_____
_____
_____.

Week 15

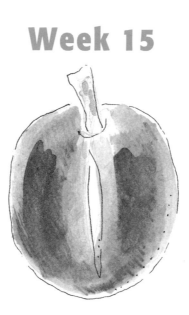

Plum

2.5 ounces

WEEK 15

I'm worried about (check what applies):
- ○ Being a good enough mother
- ○ The birth
- ○ The health of the baby
- ○ The health of our bank account
- ○ Other: _____

Physically, what's a bit weird right now is _____
_____
_____.

For exercise I am _____ _____
_____ . For stress relief, I'm _____
_____
_____.

The friend who understands me most right now is _____
_____ .

Baby, this week, your impending arrival is inspiring me to
_____
_____
_____
_____
_____
_____
_____ .

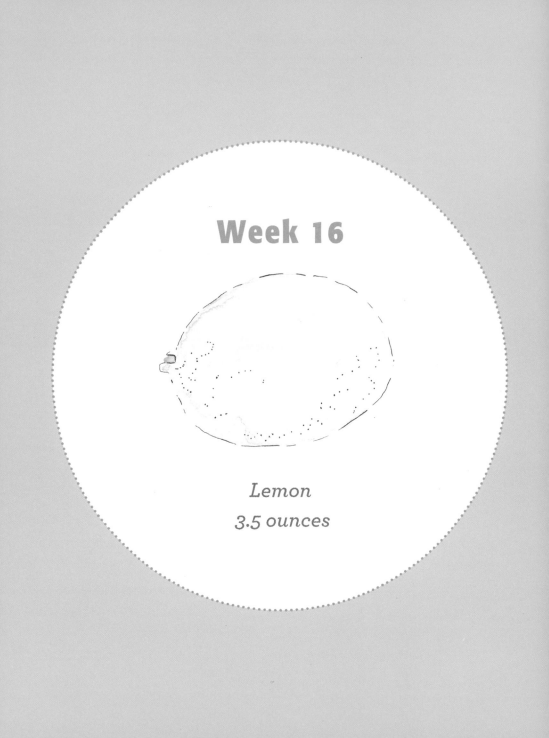

Week 16

Lemon

3.5 ounces

WEEK 16

I'm really starting to look:

- ○ Pregnant
- ○ Huge
- ○ Kind of adorable, actually
- ○ Ridiculous
- ○ Other: _____

Romance is getting really _____ right now.
Details include: _____
_____
_____ ____.

I cannot wait for the baby to one day _____
_____. When that
happens, I'm calling _____
_____ first.
Weight gain is _____ an issue for me
right now. I'm choosing to _____ _____
_____
_____.

Baby, it's so important to me that one day you have _____
_____ and _____
_____ in your life because _____
_____
_____.

Week 17

Peach

5.9 ounces

WEEK 17

Lately I've been imagining (check what applies):

- ○ Meeting this baby
- ○ The strangest things, like _____
- ○ Joining the circus
- ○ My life becoming a circus
- ○ Other: _____

My favorite baby name right now is _____.
My partner's favorite is _____. The only name
we both like/may have to agree to is _____
_____.

Wardrobe items being left behind include _____
_____
_____.

My partner is acting amazing about _____
_____. And not so
amazing about _____
_____.

Baby, I want you to grow up to be _____
_____
_____
_____
_____
_____.

Week 18

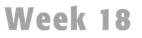

Avocado

6.7 ounces

WEEK 18

My favorite activity at the moment is (check what applies):

- ○ Napping
- ○ Shopping
- ○ Brainstorming baby names
- ○ Holding up tiny baby outfits and wondering what this baby will look like in them
- ○ Other: _____

My feeling about doing Kegels is _____
_____. The oddest place I remember to do them is _____
_____.

Childbirth classes are _____ my radar. There's a chance we will try _____
_____
_____.

In a couple words, my current plan for the birth is _____
_____
_____.

Baby, someone gave me this advice about you and I don't want to forget it: _____
_____
_____
_____.

A Pumpkin in Progress

*Use these pages to write down a story
or place a keepsake from your pregnancy so far.*

Week 19

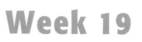

Orange

8.5 ounces

WEEK 19

Physically, what's driving me crazy this week is my (check what applies):

- ○ Skin
- ○ Back
- ○ Round ligaments (I can't believe I know what those are.)
- ○ My belly not fitting into what I want to fit it into

The thing I am NOT worried about is _____
_____.

The baby can hear now. What he/she probably hears most is
_____
_____.

My emotions this week are _____
_____
_____
_____.

Baby, I hope you always have enough _____
_____
_____
_____
_____
_____
_____.

Week 20

Tomato

10.6 ounces

WEEK 20

Halfway through! Lately, my mood is mostly (check what applies):

- ○ Celebratory
- ○ Lighthearted
- ○ Mercurial...and just the tiniest bit crazy, too
- ○ Let's face it: I'm just a big crybaby
- ○ Other: _____

Sleeping requires _____
_____.

And sometimes _____
_____.

Intimacy is _____ and involves _____
_____
_____.

We _____ finding out the sex of our baby.

In my heart, I think it's a _____.

Baby, this week, what I'm most worried about for you is that one day you'll _____
_____
_____
_____
_____.

Week 21

Bell pepper

12.7 ounces

WEEK 21

The baby's movements feel like (check what applies):
- ○ A swift kick in the bladder
- ○ Tiny bubbles
- ○ A wave
- ○ Still can't feel a thing!
- ○ Other: _____

I'm buying this baby _____.
And _____,
even though I have no idea what we are supposed to do with it.
My parents are acting _____.
And it makes me feel _____
_____.

The thing I am most excited about this week is _____
_____
_____.

Baby, I'm not perfect. Something I'm working on becoming
better for you is _____
_____
_____
_____
_____
_____
_____.

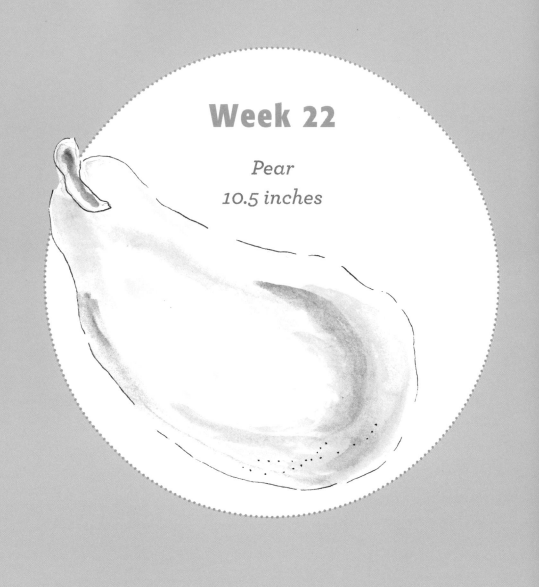

Week 22

Pear
10.5 inches

WEEK 22

When people touch my belly, it's (check what applies):

○ Nice

○ Strange—they'd better ask first

○ Constant

○ Not really an issue. I could use the extra attention.

○ Other: _____

Stretch marks are _____
_____.

When people make comments about the size of my belly, my response is _____
_____.

The one person who is driving me crazy lately is _____. Other than patience and compassion, my plan is _____
_____.

Baby, I don't expect you to be perfect. I'll support you by _____
_____
_____
_____
_____
_____
_____
_____.

Week 23

Onion

12.9 ounces

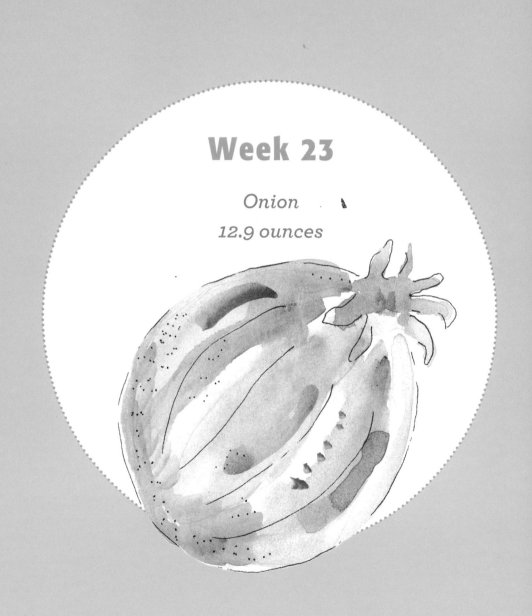

WEEK 23

Right now, exercise consists mostly of (check what applies):

○ Trips to the mailbox

○ Nice walks. A few mild workouts.

○ My normal workout

○ Not a whole lot. I'm on a break.

○ Other: _____

Lately, I've been thinking that what makes someone a good mother is _____ _____ _____.

When I'm with other people's kids, I notice _____ _____ _____ more. _____ seems so much more real now.

And _____ seems like forever ago to me.

Baby, when it comes to college someday, I hope you _____ _____ _____ _____ _____ _____.

Week 24

Sweet potato
1 pound

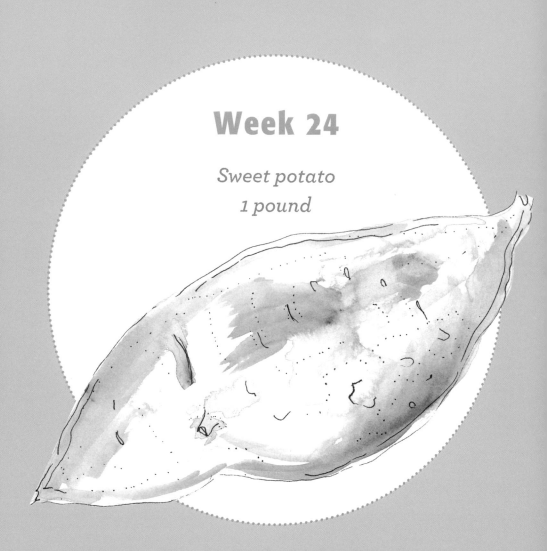

WEEK 24

When I'm on the move, I feel (check what applies):
- ○ Slow as molasses
- ○ Like a Mack truck
- ○ Sort of graceful and languid
- ○ Fertile, semi-goddess-like
- ○ Other: _____

The temperature I need right now is _____
_____.

I am wearing _____all the
time these days.

I've started thinking about the birth. When I do, I'm most
focused on _____
_____
_____
_____.

Baby, when it comes to the important things in life, more than
anything, I hope you choose _____
_____
_____
_____
_____
_____
_____.

A Pumpkin in Progress

*Use these pages to write down a story
or place a keepsake from your pregnancy so far.*

Week 25

Mango
1.5 pounds

WEEK 25

My feeling toward my partner this week is (check what applies):

- ○ Grateful. Loving. Emotional.
- ○ Hot and heavy
- ○ A bit impatient, honestly
- ○ Grumpy. Can you blame me?
- ○ Other: _____

I never realized how much I loved _____
_____.

During the day, I'm _____
_____.

At night, I'm _____
_____
_____.

My perfect meal right now is _____
_____.

Baby, I think our most important decision for you will be _____
_____
_____
_____
_____
_____
_____
_____.

Week 26

Artichoke
1.7 pounds

WEEK 26

This baby seems (check what applies):

- ○ More real than ever
- ○ Strong as a longshoreman
- ○ Bent on keeping me up all night
- ○ To not like my penchant for _____
- ○ Other: _____

The baby's room is _____
_____
_____.

My birth plan includes _____
_____. And possibly
_____.

Worst case scenario, I'm planning on _____
_____
_____.

I'm thinking _____
_____ on the epidural question.

Baby, when it comes to religion, I want you to know _____
_____
_____
_____
_____
_____.

Week 27

Rutabaga
1.8 pounds

WEEK 27

My thoughts on breast-feeding include (check what applies):

- ○ Giving it my best shot
- ○ 100% commitment
- ○ Seeing what the girls are up for
- ○ Being open to what is most sane/healthy for all
- ○ Other: _____

Some discomfort I'm having right now includes _____
_____.

The way I deal with it _____
_____.

For breakfast, I'm often in the mood for _____.

For lunch, it's _____.

And dinner is _____
_____.

My perfect day includes _____
_____.

Baby, about true love, I think _____
_____
_____
_____
_____
_____
_____
_____.

There's really a (big) baby in there.

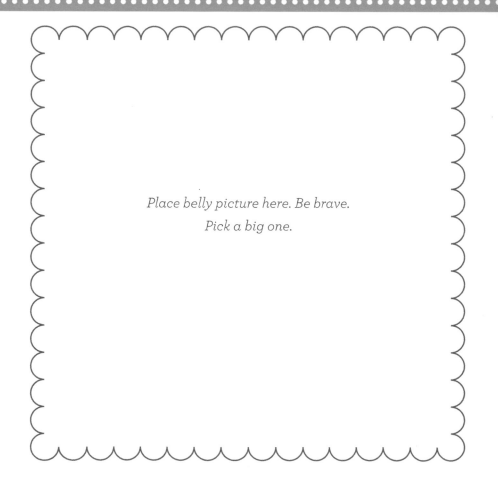

Place belly picture here. Be brave.

Pick a big one.

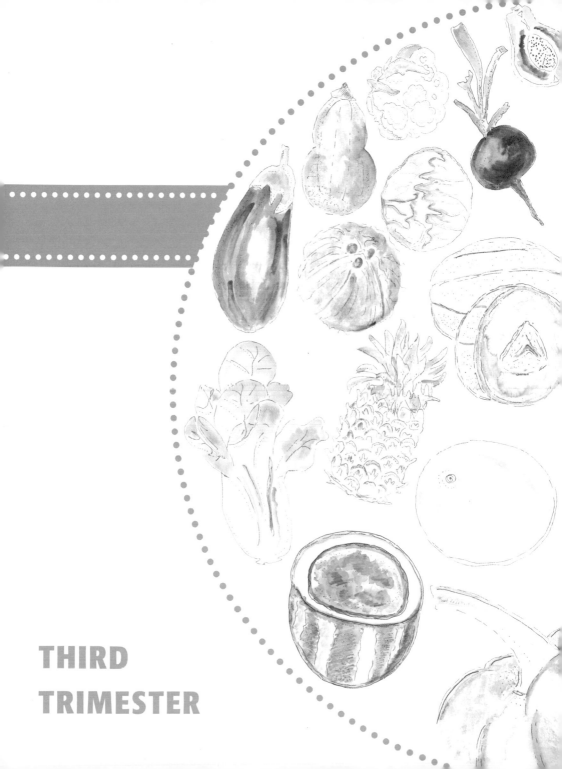

THIRD
TRIMESTER

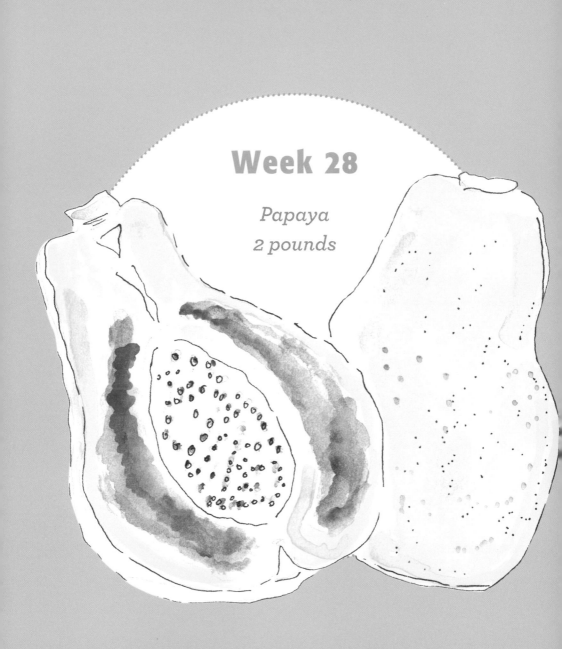

Week 28

Papaya
2 pounds

WEEK 28

In the last trimester, it's feeling like (check what applies):
- ○ This is actually going to happen
- ○ We're seeing the light at the end of the tunnel
- ○ I'm in no rush to get to the finish line
- ○ This baby will never get here
- ○ Other: _____

We want a pediatrician who is _____
_____.

The baby names on our list right now are _____
_____ and _____
_____.

This baby moves most _____
_____
_____.

Baby, there is something you should know about your parents.
We're _____
_____
_____
_____
_____
_____
_____
_____.

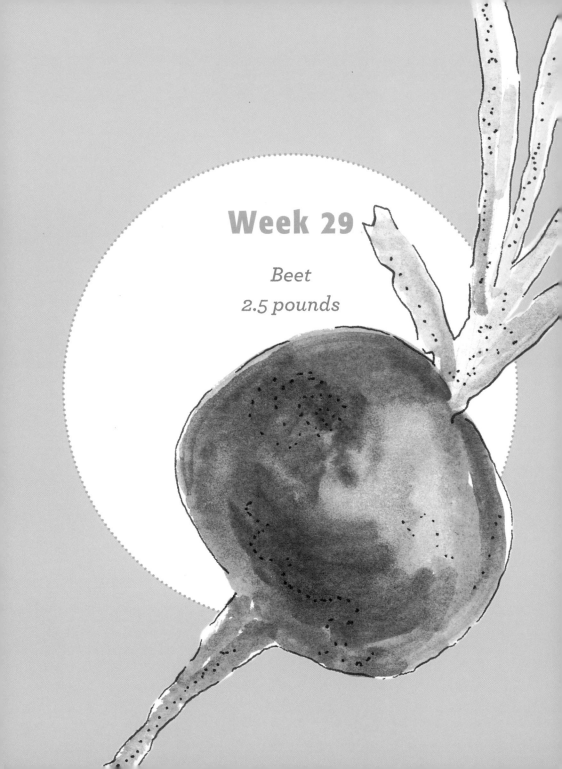

Week 29

Beet
2.5 pounds

WEEK 29

This baby kicks (check what applies):
- ○ Like he's at the World Cup
- ○ After I eat _____
- ○ Like an elegant dancer
- ○ Only at 2 a.m. or some other inopportune moment
- ○ Other: _____

For me, heartburn is _____. The pregnancy symptom challenging me the most right now is _____.

After this baby comes, I probably won't be able to _____ _____ for a while, so I'm getting it out of my system now.

My plans for the first few months after the birth include _____ _____ _____.

Baby, being our kid is going to be so _____ _____ _____ _____ _____ _____ _____ _____ _____.

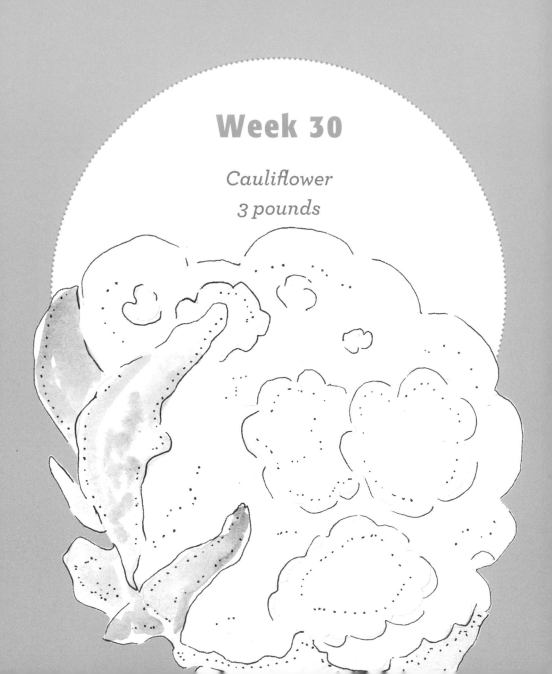

Week 30

Cauliflower
3 pounds

WEEK 30

My family is (check what applies):

- ○ Breathing down my neck
- ○ A godsend
- ○ Pretty cute about this whole preg-o thing
- ○ Not so cute. More _____
- ○ Other: _____

Something I'm really learning about my partner through this pregnancy is _____.
And that I'm kind of _____. Oh, and _____
_____ too.
I want to be the kind of mother who _____
_____
_____.

All of this baby gear makes me _____.
Especially _____ and _____
_____
_____.

Baby, I will always try to treat you _____
_____
_____
_____
_____.

Week 31

Squash
3.5 pounds

WEEK 31

What I'm packing for the birth includes (check what applies):

- ○ An inspiring photo
- ○ Good snacks
- ○ A you-will-survive-this playlist
- ○ A toothbrush and _____

What my partner did lately that saved the day was _____
_____
_____.

My wardrobe is down to _____
_____.

For the baby this week, we bought _____
_____ and _____
_____
_____
_____.

Baby, something my mom did for me that I'd like to do for you
is _____
_____
_____
_____
_____
_____
_____.

A Pumpkin in Progress

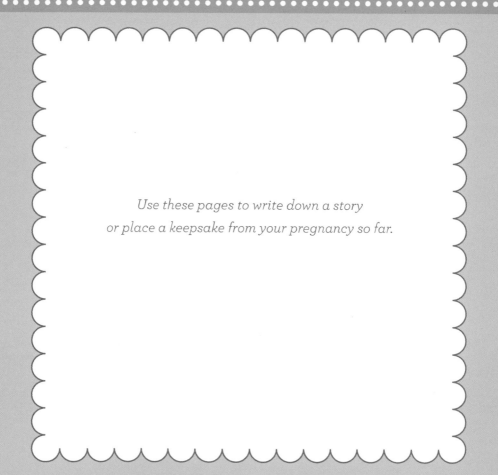

*Use these pages to write down a story
or place a keepsake from your pregnancy so far.*

Week 32

Cabbage
3.75 pounds

WEEK 32

At this point, this baby (check what applies):

- ○ Is giving me _____ of the serious kind
- ○ Appears pretty chill
- ○ Moves like James Brown
- ○ Seems exactly like _____
- ○ Other: _____

My favorite activity at the moment is _____
_____
_____ .

Something I don't miss about my pre-pregnant life that
surprises me is _____ _____
_____
_____ .

During labor, I want so badly to _____
_____ and I think it will help
if I _____
_____ .

Baby, if your friends let you down someday, as people
sometimes do, remember _____
_____
_____
_____
_____ .

Week 33

Coconut
4.2 pounds

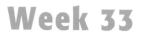

WEEK 33

My walk lately is (check what applies):

- ○ More of a waddle
- ○ Just a walk. I still got it.
- ○ Not happening. I'm mostly sitting and lying about.
- ○ Completely normal
- ○ Other: _____

The time I feel most connected to this baby is _____
_____
_____.

I keep daydreaming about _____
_____
_____ with the baby someday.

The first thing I will do when I meet this baby is _____
_____
_____.

Baby, I hope the way you handle yourself in the world one day
will be mostly _____
_____
_____
_____
_____
_____
_____
_____.

Week 34

Eggplant
4.75 pounds

WEEK 34

Fatigue lately is (check what applies):

○ A non-issue

○ Debilitating

○ Directly related to the time of day

○ Eased by chocolate or foot rubs

○ Other: _____

Speaking of foot rubs, the other thing that really helps me right now is _____
_____.

I think the biggest adjustment when this baby arrives will be
_____
_____
_____. Or maybe _____
_____
_____.

Everyone tells me to sleep now. My sleep is _____
_____
_____ at the moment.

Baby, I hope your hair is _____
_____
_____. Just like your _____
_____
_____.

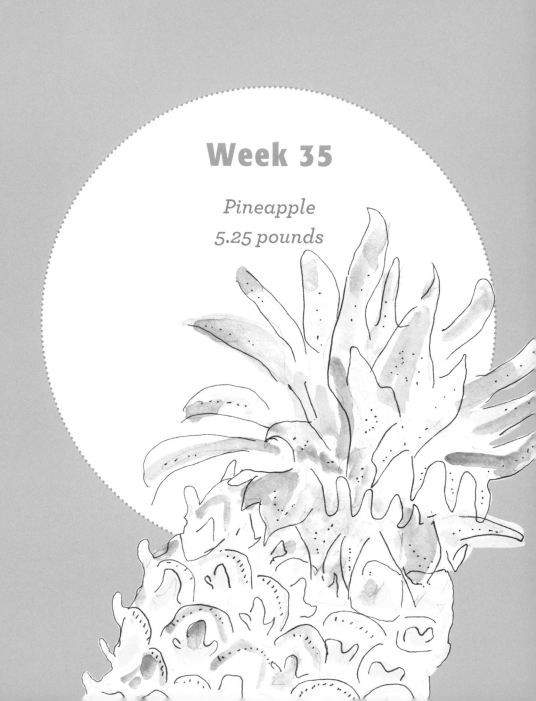

Week 35

Pineapple
5.25 pounds

WEEK 35

My outlook on the baby's arrival is (check what applies):

○ Beyond ecstatic

○ Scared, excited

○ A nervous wreck

○ Pretty blissed out. And more than ready.

○ Other: _____

My belly is _____

_____

_____.

I hope I never forget _____

_____

_____

_____ about this pregnancy.

We still need _____

_____

_____.

Baby, I promise not to _____

_____

_____

_____

_____

_____

_____.

Week 36

Cantaloupe
5.8 pounds

WEEK 36

My dietary choices of late include (check what applies):

○ Not much to be proud of

○ Mostly healthy, with a little touch of _____ and _____

○ Almost all _____, especially at _____

○ More budget than gourmet

○ Other: _____

The first person I want called about this baby's arrival is_____
_____.

The class we took or book we read that was the most helpful was _____
_____.

I'm relieved about _____
_____. My partner is relieved about _____
and worried about _____
_____.

Baby, someday, I plan on telling you all about _____
_____
_____
_____
_____.

Week 37

Honeydew
6.2 pounds

WEEK 37

People say I'm carrying this baby (check what applies):
- ○ High
- ○ Low
- ○ Like I swallowed a basketball
- ○ Like I swallowed a really large, wide basketball
- ○ Other: _____

When I lay awake at night, I think about _____
_____.

My plan for the first few weeks after the baby comes is _____
_____.

And I want _____ with me.

And _____
_____.

The due date is approaching and all I can think about is _____
_____
_____.

Baby, I am already proud of your _____
_____
_____
_____
_____
_____
_____.

A Pumpkin in Progress

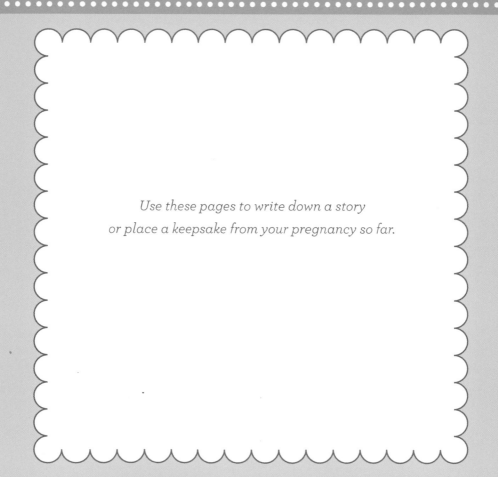

*Use these pages to write down a story
or place a keepsake from your pregnancy so far.*

Week 38

Baby bok choi
6.5 pounds

WEEK 38

There is still (check what applies):

- ○ A lot to do
- ○ A lot to worry about
- ○ A lot to be anxious about
- ○ A lot to be happy about

In preparation for this baby, I'm brushing up on my _____
_____ skills. And stockpiling
_____
and _____
_____.

I wonder, will the baby _____
_____?

This baby's personality seems to be _____
_____
_____
_____.

Baby, I can't wait to _____
_____
_____
_____
_____
_____
_____.

Week 39

Watermelon
7.25 pounds

WEEK 39

The birth seems (check what applies):
- ○ Imminent
- ○ Like it's going to happen to someone else
- ○ Like it might be slightly comedic
- ○ Totally real
- ○ Other: _____

I'm getting better at _____
_____
_____.

I think I've learned to be more _____
_____
_____.

I hope I never forget how my partner _____
_____
_____ during this pregnancy. And how
_____
_____ it made me feel.

Baby, the truth is _____
_____
_____
_____
_____
_____.

Week 40

Pumpkin
7.5 pounds

WEEK 40

At this point, my feeling about being pregnant is (check what applies):

- ○ Done. But nervous about the next step.
- ○ Totally ready to not be
- ○ I'll miss it
- ○ Already planning my sushi and beer post-pregnancy dinner
- ○ Other:_____

Before the baby comes, we still need _____
_____
_____.

If labor could just not _____
_____
_____.

The outfit this baby is wearing on Day One is _____
_____
_____
_____.

Baby, you are already _____
_____
_____
_____.

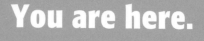

You are here.

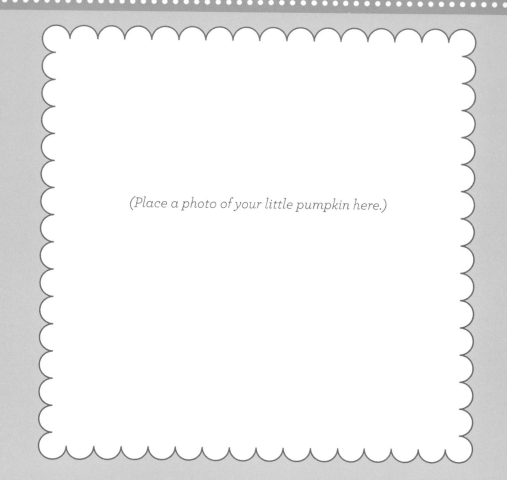

(Place a photo of your little pumpkin here.)

THE BIRTH

Labor and delivery were (check what applies):

- ○ What I expected
- ○ Nothing that I expected
- ○ The hardest thing I've ever done
- ○ Not so tough. We're already talking about a brother or sister.

The baby's name is _____

_____.

It's a _____ and

(circle one) he/she looks kind of/exactly like _____

_____

_____.

Baby, I had no idea I would _____

_____

_____

_____

_____.

I am so _____

_____.

I will never forget _____

_____

_____

_____.

ABOUT THE AUTHOR/ ILLUSTRATOR

Geralyn Broder Murray is a writer of advertising, books, and other things that make people happy/buy stuff/do stuff. She began drawing at age forty. Find her online at www.BigShotWriter.com.

For more on *From Pea to Pumpkin,* go to www.PeaToPumpkin.com. "Like" us on Facebook for regular P2P updates throughout your pregnancy and beyond.